Egg Cookbook

2nd Edition

A Collection of 25 Delicious, Quick & Tasty Egg Recipes for Breakfast, Lunch & Dinner

by Olivia Rogers

Copyright © 2017 By Olivia Rogers
All rights reserved. No part of this book may be reproduced in any form without permission in writing from the author. No part of this publication may be reproduced or transmitted in any form or by any means, mechanic, electronic, photocopying, recording, by any storage or retrieval system, or transmitted by email without the permission in writing from the author and publisher.
For information regarding permissions write to author at
Olivia@TheMenuAtHome.com
Reviewers may quote brief passages in review.

Please note that credit for the images used in this book go to the respective owners. You can view this at: TheMenuAtHome.com/image-list

Olivia Rogers
TheMenuAtHome.com

Table of Contents

Introduction	5
1. Scalloped Eggs	8
2. Biscuit Sandwich	10
3. Migas	12
4. Greek Family Omelet	14
5. Eggs in Purgatory	16
6. Moroccan Eggs	18
7. Nicoise Deviled Eggs	20
8. Ham Frittata	22
9. Swiss Chard and Cheddar Quiche	24
10. Friseé with Bacon and Soft Cooked Eggs	26
11. Egg Pizza	28
12. Deconstructed Croque Madame	31
13. Eggs Florentine	34
14. Egg Spaghetti	37
15. Lemon Chile Rigatoni with Grated Egg Yolk	39
16. Local Egg Noodle Casserole	41

17. Delicious Pasta	43
18. Mexican Huevos Rancheros	45
19. Menemen aka Istanbul's Breakfast	47
20. Tuscany Pastured Eggs	49
21. Chinese Egg Drop Soup	51
22. Avocado Egg Salad	53
23. Hummus Egg Salad	55
24. Pork Egg Salad	57
25. Beef Egg Salad	59
Final Words	61
Disclaimer	62

Introduction

Eggs. Used to be a staple in the English or American breakfast standards. Scrambled, omelet, cooked whichever way you prefer.

Especially during Easter, everyone thinks of eggs in almost any other way thinkable. Chocolate, jelly, colorfully decorated (especially red) hard boiled eggs, etc.

For some reason, recently, people have reduced the consumption of eggs not just during breakfast but in general. At some point there was even a general medical recommendation not to eat more than a specific number of eggs per day.

That's just it!

Over a specific number! Not take eggs out of the dietary habits altogether! Here are ten health related reasons, to re-introduce eggs into your diet:

1. The carotenoid content of one egg per day may prevent macular degeneration.

2. Further benefits of carotenoid ingredients zeaxanthin and lutein refer to reducing the risk of developing cataracts.

3. All 9 essential amino acids and 6 grams of protein are ingested upon eating just one egg.

4. Contrary to the previous beliefs that eggs are linked with heart disease, studies conducted at Harvard School of Public health proved that eating eggs regularly may prevent blood clots, heart attacks and strokes.

5. Just one egg yolk contains 300 microgram of choline which is a nutrient used to regulate the nervous system, the brain and the cardiovascular system.

6. The belief that eggs are high in fat is correct, but it is the correct fat.

7. The aforementioned medical recommendation for a certain number of eggs per day was based on initial studies that showed increased levels of cholesterol. Further studies corrected the initial assumption and stipulated that moderate consumption does not actually affect cholesterol. 2 eggs per day may even improve the lipid profile.

8. It is the only natural food that contains Vitamin D.

9. Consuming 6 eggs per week lowers the risk of breast cancer considerably. The relevant study revealed a percentage of 44%.

10. Especially for women the high sulfuric content along with the minerals and vitamins provided, promotes the health of hair and nails.

At this point it should be mentioned that all the above references, in no way intend to replace the advice and consultation provided by your own personal physician. In fact, it is strongly recommended to seek such advice and guidance before including more eggs than necessary in your diet. There may be other underlying medical conditions involved that may be adversely affected.

For some people, taking the eggs out of the dietary habits was a matter of bad taste. Keep reading, and it is certain that you will reconsider. You may have gotten full of eating eggs the same way over and over again, but there are plenty of recipes to test.

Some of them have been included in this e-book. There are plenty more online. And, of course, you can always experiment on your own until you find a set that will be to your personal liking.

However, it is important that eggs return to your table. They are too valuable for your own health to keep leaving them out. If you really want to enjoy a little better quality of life than the one you have now, foods like eggs must be in the plate in front of you as many times per week as your doctor tells you. It's as simple as that.

1. Scalloped Eggs

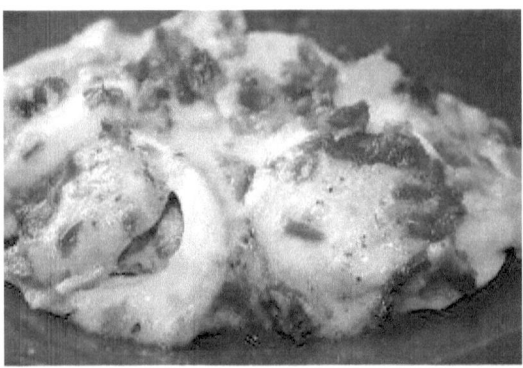

Taking the subject one level higher, it's time to start introducing egg dishes. Remember that we are trying to persuade people that do not like the taste of eggs to still include them in their diet. Cheating the taste a bit is not a great crime in the big picture of good health.

Ingredients

- 2 boiled potatoes, sliced
- 4 eggs
- 6 tablespoons of milk
- 6 tablespoons of sour cream
- 1 tablespoon flour

Method

1. Hard cook the eggs and slice them. Take a baking dish, butter it and layer the eggs and the potatoes. Season with nutmeg, salt and pepper to taste.

2. Whisk the milk, the sour cream and the flour over the layers. Top with breadcrumbs. Cook at 350°F for 25 minutes.

Potatoes

This recipe is a good choice to feed children who do not seem to be able to eat any food without potatoes. Many parents feel that eating potatoes that much is not good. On the contrary, a medium size potato contains high fiber, vitamins A, C, D, E, K, the entire complex of vitamin B, choline and betaine.

Therefore, it's not just nutritious. It's another superfood. So, with this dish, you are actually feeding your children (and yourself) with enough protection against many ailments, heart conditions, disorders and a multitude of other medical conditions that would have cost you a rather steep amount of money to the doctors and hospitals, if and when such time ever came.

2. Biscuit Sandwich

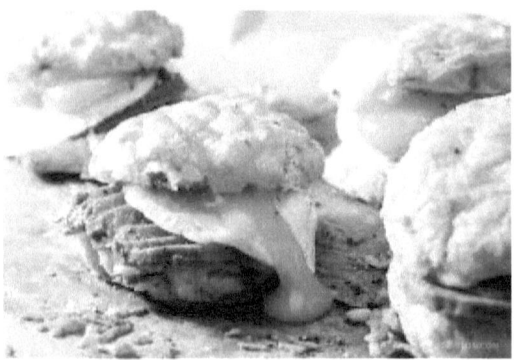

This is supposed to be a children party special, but just by reading about it, most adults would want to at least try it. It combines quite a few tasty things and is nutritious too.

Ingredients

- 2 eggs
- 1 tablespoon chopped chives
- Cheddar
- Cooked sausage patty

Method

1. Scramble the eggs (everyone knows how to do that) adding the chives. Take a biscuit and split it in two halves.

2. Take the first half melt a slice of cheddar, add the sausage patty and the eggs and top with the other half.

Tips

This is a CHILDREN's PARTY SPECIAL. Please leave some for the children (it is guaranteed that once you taste this, you will not stop eating it).

3. Migas

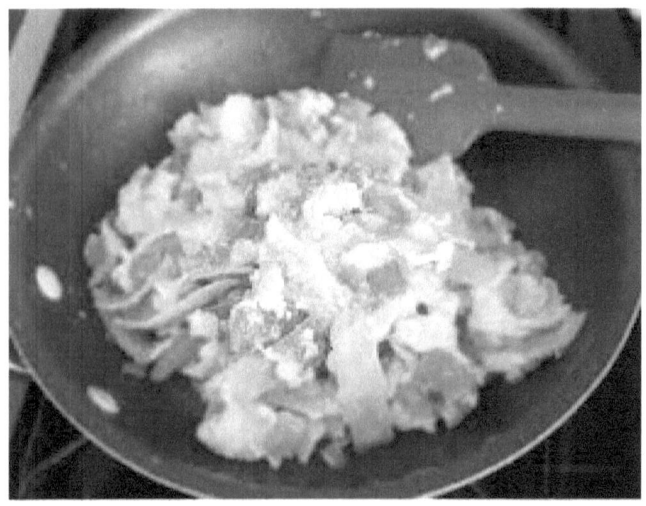

Time to start speaking a bit of Spanish. You've been speaking burritos and tortillas anyway. Time to speak migas as well. Well... speaking may be a bit of an overstatement... Probably after having this dish you'll be speechless.

Ingredients

- 4 tortillas
- 5 eggs
- Grated cheddar
- ½ cup sliced onion
- Roasted poblano peppers
- Vegetable oil
- Salsa
- Cilantro

Method

1. Make sure that the tortillas are thinly sliced and use the vegetable oil to sauté for 5 minutes in a skillet with the onion and the peppers.

2. Beat the eggs and introduce them to the skillet. Stir until the eggs are set. Top with the cheddar and the rest of the ingredients.

Tips

Vegetable oil, eggs and cheese. This combination is recommended in almost every diet that is suggested by dieticians and nutritionists worldwide. Why? Because it has all the necessary ingredients to make it a dish to control your weight and get protection from bacteria and other harmful agents.

4. Greek Family Omelet

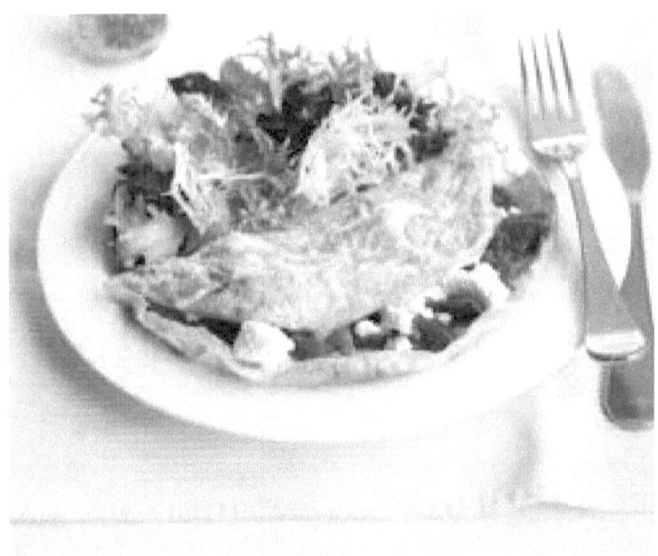

Spinach, asparagus, fruit and other omelets have been a dietary staple for decades. Time to discuss a piece of the Mediterranean diet. Since we are learning to speak multiple languages here, it seems like a very good idea.

Ingredients

- 8 eggs (or 2 for each member of the family)
- Olive oil
- 2 tablespoons of milk
- Diced ham
- Gruyere or feta cheese
- Sliced potatoes
- Tomato paste

Method

1. Cut the potatoes to French fry size and put in a frying pan and start frying with olive oil. Take the eggs and beat them in a separate bowl. Season with salt and pepper to taste.

2. If you use gruyere make sure it's well grated. If you use feta, make sure it's cut to small cubes. Introduce the cheese to the bowl with the eggs and mix very well. Then introduce the tomato paste and the diced ham and keep mixing until the mixture is well-balanced.

3. About 5 minutes before the potatoes are ready, pour the mix evenly into the frying pan. Let the bottom set but not brown.

4. The traditional Greek way requires to take another frying pan, put it on top and with an abrupt and very fast move turn the omelet upside down and cook the other side too. If you cannot do that, fold the omelet like a letter.

Tips

In the other recipes we discussed about putting one or two superfoods together. This one has four. It is strongly recommended that you do not mix this dish with other ones. An overload of nutrients may be just as dangerous as a diet that lacks them.

5. Eggs in Purgatory

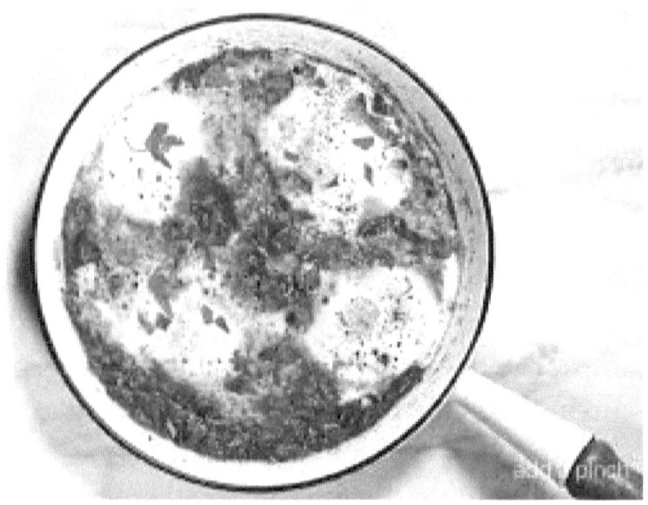

The title doesn't sound right until you take a look at the ingredients and see how easy it is to make. It could make for a very nice side dish, or a very nutritious breakfast on its own.

Ingredients

- Marinara sauce
- 6 eggs
- Parmesan

Method

1. Take a small baking dish and pour in the sauce until it is half full. Crack the eggs and throw them in. Back for 10 to 12 minutes at 350°F. Whisk parmesan on top.

Tips

This is a very unique taste. And very Italian. I.e. the journey around the world continues...

6. Moroccan Eggs

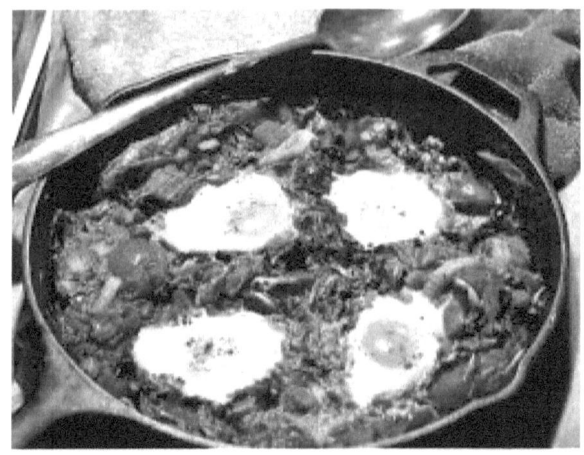

This is another style of Mediterranean diet. Still with olive oil but with enough spice to make your nostrils flame out. (No, this is not a Game of Thrones dragon primer...)

Ingredients

- 6 eggs
- 1 cup chickpeas
- Marinara sauce
- Paprika
- Ground cumin

Method

1. Take an ovenproof skillet and toast with some olive oil the chickpeas, cumin and paprika. Fill the skillet with marinara sauce.

2. Take the eggs and crack them in. Bake at 350°F for 10 to 12 minutes or until the egg whites are firm

Tips

People all over the world have been using eggs in their cooking recognizing their great value. Each different kind of people has its own recipes and its own procedures on making very tasty dishes that can stand out.

If you want to have an informed opinion about eggs, you simply must taste them all. You may become bored, but you will probably be the healthiest person on earth. And that should count for something...

7. Nicoise Deviled Eggs

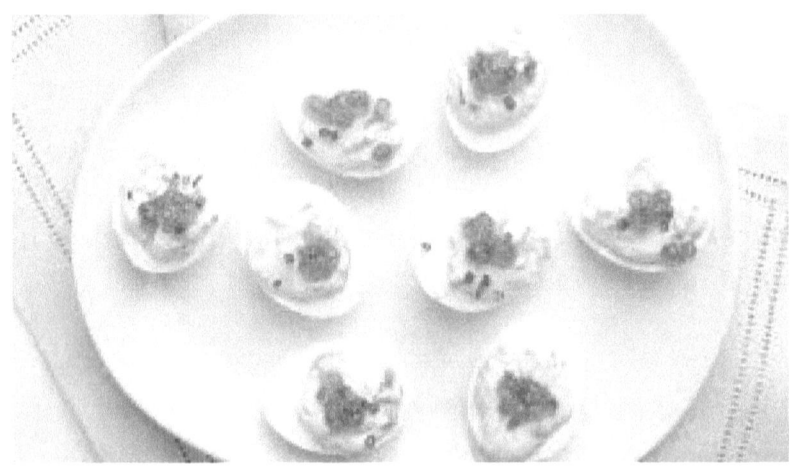

Time to go to Cyprus and Nicosia. It is also time to begin introducing more anti-oxidants and omega 3 fatty acids to the equation of the necessary nutrients to the human body.

Ingredients

- Eggs (2 per person to be served)
- 3 tablespoons olive oil
- Tuna
- Sliced olives
- Tomatoes

Method

1. Hard cook the eggs, cut in halves and take out the yolks. Take a bowl and mash the olive oil, a can of tuna, some chopped parsley and some lemon juice.

2. Scoop the mash into the egg whites and top with the tomatoes and the olives.

Tips

This is one of the fastest recipes available. It can be ready for breakfast within 7 minutes, 8 tops. This will give you no more excuses to skip breakfast because you just woke up and there is no time to prepare a proper breakfast before you go to work, or sent the kids to school.

Breakfast is always the most important meal of the day. Ask any doctor you like, and they will tell you the same thing. And it is one of the most important mistakes made in the western diet.

8. Ham Frittata

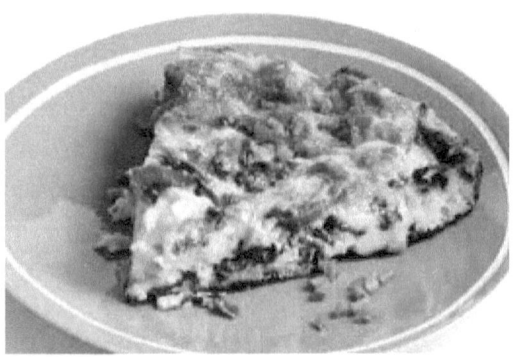

The previous recipe was a fast one. This is a slow one. However, it is also one of the tastier ones that you will find. It does have a lot of ingredients but from all accounts, it will be well worth the effort to cook it and then enjoy it. Slowly please...

Ingredients

- 8 eggs
- 3 ounces diced ham
- ½ cup milk
- 1 cup sliced asparagus
- ¾ cup shredded pecorino

Method

1. Beat the eggs, pecorino, milk with as much salt and pepper as you want. Sauté the asparagus and the ham in a skillet with olive oil.

2. Add the egg mixture and cook until the bottom sets. Bake for 25 minutes at 325°F

Asparagus

The body does not need only amino acids, vitamins, proteins, carbs and fat. It also needs minerals like copper, manganese, phosphorus, potassium, zinc and iron. You will not easily find another food that contains as many minerals as asparagus.

In the usual manner of the superfoods, it also contains vitamins C, E, B2, B6 and K, fiber, niacin and pantothenic acid. If this all sound Greek or Chinese to you, your doctor will gladly let you know what these are all about.

9. Swiss Chard and Cheddar Quiche

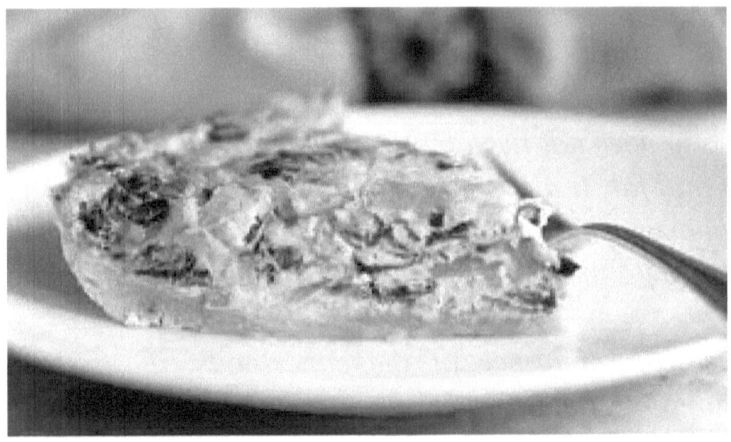

Time to take the recipes one step further. The following dish requires 15 minutes preparation and a total of an hour to cook. It is a dish very rich in calcium and properly balanced in reference to carbohydrates, fat and protein.

Ingredients

- 3 tablespoons of olive oil
- 1 tablespoon vinegar from red wine
- 1 chopped onion
- 3 eggs
- 1 9-inch prebaked piecrust
- ¾ cup half-and-half
- Kosher salt and pepper
- ½ cup of grated cheddar
- 4 cups lettuce
- 1 bunch chopped Swiss chard

Method

1. Preheat your oven to 350°F. Take a large skillet, heat one of the tablespoons of the olive oil in medium heat and add the onion and the chard. Cook for 3 to 4 minutes.

2. Take a bowl and beat the eggs with the half-and-half. Season with salt and pepper. Add the chard and the cheddar and mix. Pour onto the piecrust and bake for 40 to 45 minutes or until it sets.

3. Waiting for the baking process to be completed, use another medium bowl to mix the lettuce, the vinegar and the rest of the oil to prepare a green salad. Season with salt and pepper. Serve when it's ready in a dish with the salad on the side.

Tips

This dish contains 10 grams of saturated fat, 226 calories, 133 mg cholesterol, 813 mg of sodium, 9 grams of protein, 23 grams of carbohydrate, 3 grams of sugar, 152 mg of calcium, 2 mg of iron and 1-gram fiber.

If you are ever on a diet counting the intake, these numbers will be very useful to you.

10. Friseé with Bacon and Soft Cooked Eggs

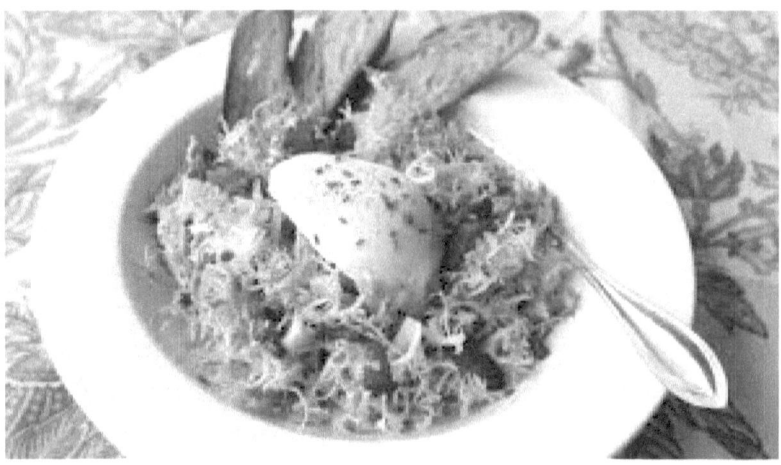

Time for dinner. All doctors will tell you that dinner should be a light meal and that it should be consumed quite some time before going to bed. Therefore, it has to be a dish that will not allow you to go sit on the couch and start dipping on snacks.

Spending 25 minutes on this dish will make it so.

Ingredients

- 8 eggs
- 3 tablespoons vinegar from red wine
- 4 cups torn friseé
- 4 slices of bacon
- 1 tablespoon of olive oil
- 4 cups of torn radicchio

Method

1. Pour some water in a medium saucepan and bring it to boil. Add the eggs very gently and boil for 6 minutes. Afterwards, rinse the eggs under cold water and peel them.

2. Cook the bacon in medium heat in a large skillet for 7 to 9 minutes or until it is crisp. Afterwards remove it, crumble it and set it aside. Add olive oil and vinegar to the bacon drippings and stir.

3. Gate a medium bowl and put in the radicchio, the friseé and the warm dressing. Toss to mix. Put the eggs and the bacon pieces on top and serve, seasoning with pepper.

Tips

The ingredients refer to dinner for at least 4 people. Please leave some for the others sharing your dinner, or leave some of it for tomorrow evening as well. The temptation to eat it all at once may be too much, but you should restrain yourself.

11. Egg Pizza

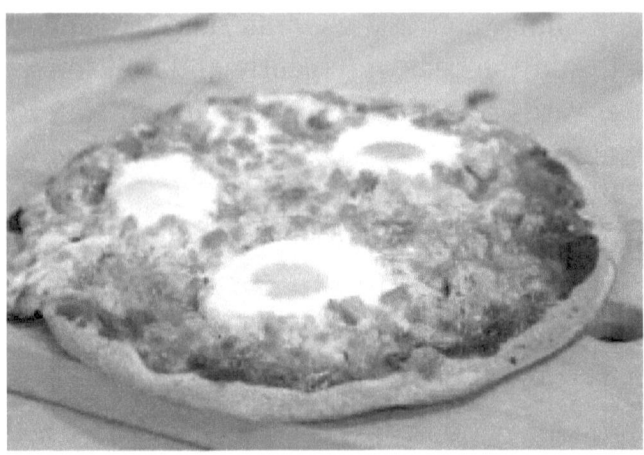

Who said that pizza had to be fattening, full of MSG, gluten and in the end bad for your health? Time to change your mind over this and definitely add pizza to your evening meals. Because there is such a thing as a healthy pizza.

Ingredients

For the dough

- ½ cup warm water
- 2 teaspoons olive oil
- ½ teaspoon salt
- About 150 grams of bread flour
- 1 teaspoon of active dry yeast

For the topping

- 3 tablespoons of olive oil

- 2 dried pepperoncini
- Fresh grated mozzarella
- 2 to 3 large eggs
- 5 garlic cloves

Method

1. Take a bowl put the water and sprinkle the yeast. Whisk until the yeast is dissolved. Cover the bowl and put it in a warm place for 5 minutes. Add the olive oil, salt and half the quantity of bread flour. Use a wooden spoon and stir for 5 minutes to form the wet dough.

2. Spread the rest of the flour on your work bench and place the wet dough on top. Start kneading and keep it up for 8 minutes or until the dough is sticky. Get a large bowl and coat the sides with olive oil. Put the dough in, in the form of a ball. Roll it around to get coated in the olive oil. Cover the bowl with a towel (damp) and put in a warm place for an hour to rise.

3. Preheat the oven to 450°F and place a rack at the lower third. Peel the garlic cloves and mash them. Take 3 of them and mix them with the olive oil. Set aside. Take a pizza peel or a baking pan and spread cornmeal. Push the dough to make a small round. Cover the pan and set aside for 20 minutes.

4. Use this time to take a saucepan heat some olive oil and crush the pepperoncino. Introduce the remaining garlic cloves into the oil with the pepperoncino and sauté for a minute. Add the tomato paste and loosen it with 1-2

tablespoons of water. Stir to mix. Take the saucepan out of the stovetop and set it aside.

5. Uncover the dough, press to form its final shape and spread the sauce, cheeses and two cracked eggs. Put it on a baking sheet and bake for 12 minutes at the lower third of the oven. Should you have a pizza stone available, transfer the pizza to the stone after 8 minutes of cooking. Bake until the crust is golden, take out and brush the exposed crust with the garlic oil right away.

Tips

There is such a thing as a healthy pizza, but no one said that it would be a snap to cook it. But as the saying goes, nothing that is worth doing is ever easy. It's time to think pretty hard if you prefer the pizza parlors and their MSG and gluten over a nice home made one.

By the way, you could also experiment a bit on this recipe and add a few materials like bacon and ham or mushrooms. Just some tweaking from your part and it will taste much better than what you will get from a pizza parlor.

12. Deconstructed Croque Madame

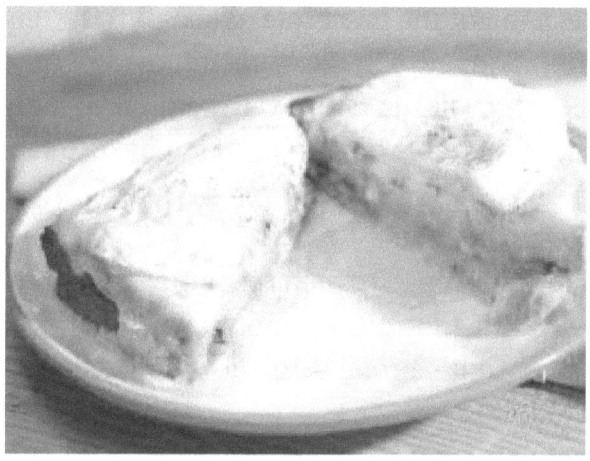

For the last recipe we have reserved the child of a casserole and a grilled cheese sandwich. For those immersed in cooking a Croque Madame is a Croque Monsieur with an egg on top. For the uninitiated it's all French. So, let's make it simple.

Ingredients

- 2 to 3 eggs
- A day-old brioche loaf 5 cups worth, cut in cubes
- 1¾ cups of cooked diced ham
- ¾ cups of milk
- 3 tablespoons of flour
- ¾ cup grated parmesan
- 1½ cups of grated gruyere
- 2 cups of half and half
- 1 tablespoon of canola oil
- 3 tablespoons butter

Method

1. Take a medium casserole dish, put the cubed bread inside, pour the milk and set aside. In a medium saucepan cook the ham over medium to high heat until it gets a golden-brown color. Set it aside too.

2. Preheat the oven to 400°F. You will need another medium saucepan to melt the butter in, add the flour and whisk until the mix is smooth. Add half and half and whisk until it's brought to a low boil. Allow a minute or two to thicken.

3. Add the cheeses and stir until the mix is smooth. Remove from heat and season with salt pepper and nutmeg. Place the ham on top of the bread and pour ¾ of the cheese mixture. Stir to mix thoroughly. Taste what you did and if necessary, use the rest of the cheese mixture.

4. Bake for 10 to 15 minutes until it's brown on top. Meanwhile take a medium saucepan and heat a tablespoon of oil until it's hot, in medium to high heat. Add the eggs gently and cook until the white is done but the yolk is still intact. This should take about three minutes. Take the casserole out of the oven, top with the eggs and serve immediately

Tips

The language lesson ended with a French touch. It's not expected that you became fluent with all the languages we

presented, but with some practice, you will learn to speak all of them.

13. Eggs Florentine

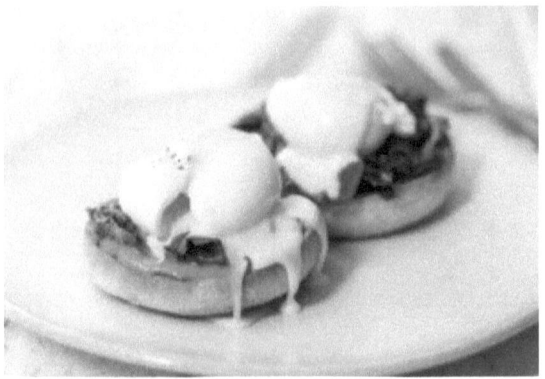

A variation of Eggs Benedicts but this dish substitutes bacon with spinach. The secret to the success of this recipe lies in the sauce. It needs to cook slowly and gently.

Serves: 4
Preparation Time: 55 minutes

Ingredients

- Hollandaise sauce
- 4 egg yolks
- 2 tbsp. fresh lime and lemon juice
- 1 tbsp. cold water
- 1/8 tsp salt
- 2 pinches white pepper (freshly ground)
- Pinch cayenne pepper
- Eggs Florentine
- 2 sticks unsalted butter (melted)
- 4 white English muffins (split, toasted)

- 3 tsp unsalted butter (softened)
- 4 cups loosely packed baby spinach leaves
- 8 medium eggs

Method

1. **To make the sauce:** Set a large heatproof bowl over a saucepan of water, barely simmering. Make sure that the base of the bowl is larger than the saucepan and therefore does not touch the water in the pan.

2. In the heatproof bowl combine the egg yolks, lime and lemon juice, and cold water. Whisk continually until the mixture thickens. Continue to whisk for a further minute, making sure to remove the bowl from the pan immediately when you see it thickening. Season with salt, pepper and cayenne.

3. Use an aerator attached to a hand blender and blend the mixture, while at the same time gently pouring the sticks of melted butter in a fine stream. It should take about 2-3 minutes for the mixtures to be incorporated. Taste and season as needed. Cover and keep the sauce warm on a very low heat until you are ready to serve.

4. Spread a thin layer of butter (2 teaspoons in total) on both sides of each muffin.

5. In a frying pan on a medium heat, melt 1 teaspoon of butter. Add the spinach to the pan and fry until it wilts slightly, about 2-3 minutes. Keep the spinach warm.

6. Add ½" cold water to an egg poaching pan, and on a medium heat bring to a slow simmer. Spray the cups with cooking spray and carefully break an egg into each greased cup. Cover the pan and poach until the whites are formed and yolks glazed but still runny, this should take around 3-4 minutes depending on your preference.

7. Transfer the cooked eggs to a warm dinner plate and repeat until all the eggs have been used.

8. Lay 2 buttered muffin halves on 4 dinner plates. Top the base of each muffin with spinach, a poached egg and hollandaise sauce. Serve immediately!

14. Egg Spaghetti

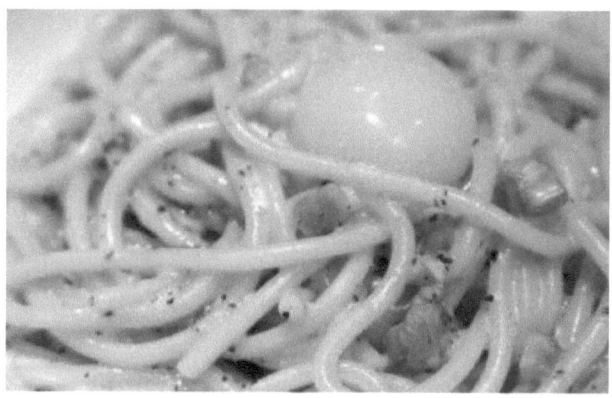

If you feel like you are lacking in vitamins, then this is full meal for you to have during the day.

Serves: 2
Preparation Time: 15 minutes

Ingredients

- Asparagus – 2
- Onion(chopped) – 1
- Garlic cloves(chopped) – 2
- Fresh herbs – 2 tbsp.
- Lemon juice – 2 tbsp.
- Butter – 2 tbsp.
- Breadcrumbs – 2 cups
- Spaghetti – 1 pack
- Eggs – 4

Method

1. Boil the spaghetti and keep aside when done. Add butter into the pot and cook on low heat.

2. Add asparagus, onion, garlic, herbs, lemon juice, breadcrumbs and eggs.

3. Cook for 10 minutes. When ready, mix both spaghetti and mixture to enjoy.

15. Lemon Chile Rigatoni with Grated Egg Yolk

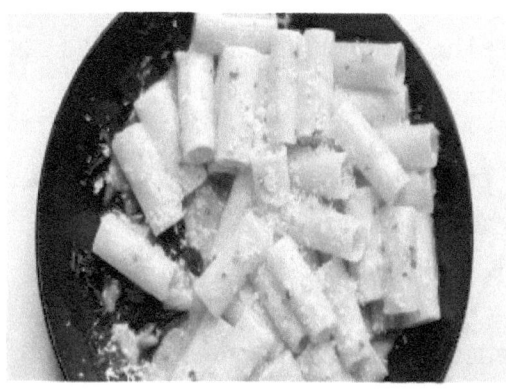

Yes, you really can grate egg yolks! And what's more, they're the perfect garnish for buttery lemon chile rigatoni.

Serves: 4
Preparation Time: 25 minutes

Ingredients

- Sea salt
- 12 ounces dried rigatoni
- 4 large hardboiled eggs
- 8 tbsp. butter
- 2 tsp lemon zest (grated)
- 4 tbsp. freshly squeezed lemon juice
- ½ tsp red Chile pepper flakes (crushed)
- Black pepper (to taste)
- ½ cup Pecorino cheese (grated)

Method

1. Salt a large pot of water and bring to a boil. Toss in the rigatoni and cook until very al dente. In the meantime, separate the yolks from the hard-boiled eggs and discard the whites.

2. Gently grate the yolks into a small bowl and set aside. Drain the pasta into a bowl, setting aside 1½ cups of the cooking water.

3. In a skillet over med-high heat, melt ¾ of the butter and sauté the lemon zest, juice and crushed red pepper flakes. Add the pasta to the skillet along with the reserved cooking water. Cook for 4-5 minutes until the sauce thickens.

4. Season with black pepper and extra salt if necessary. Sprinkle the cheese over the pasta and add in the remaining butter.

5. Toss until the cheese and butter melt and coat the pasta. Spoon the pasta evenly into warmed bowls and finish with a sprinkle of grated egg yolk. Enjoy!

16. Local Egg Noodle Casserole

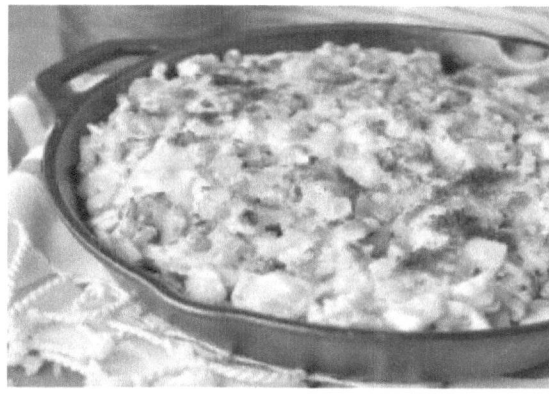

At less than 500 calories per serving, this casserole is a great way to enjoy a nutritious and healthy meal.

Serves: 4
Preparation Time: 40 minutes

Ingredients

- 3 cups dry broad egg noodles (cooked)
- 2 cups pasta sauce
- 1 cup low fat cottage cheese
- 8 eggs (hardboiled, peeled, sliced)
- 1 cup low-fat mozzarella cheese (grated)
- 2 tbsp. fresh Parmesan cheese (grated)

Method

1. Preheat the main oven to 350 F. Lightly coat a 2-quart casserole dish with cooking spray. Add 1½ cups of

cooked noodles, 1 cup of pasta sauce, ½ cup of cottage cheese, ½ of the sliced egg and ½ cup of grated mozzarella to the dish.

2. Repeat the layer. Scatter Parmesan cheese over the top of the casserole and completely cover with foil.

3. Transfer to the preheated oven and bake for 15 minutes. Remove the foil and cook for a further 10-12 minutes, until the cheese is bubbling.

17. Delicious Pasta

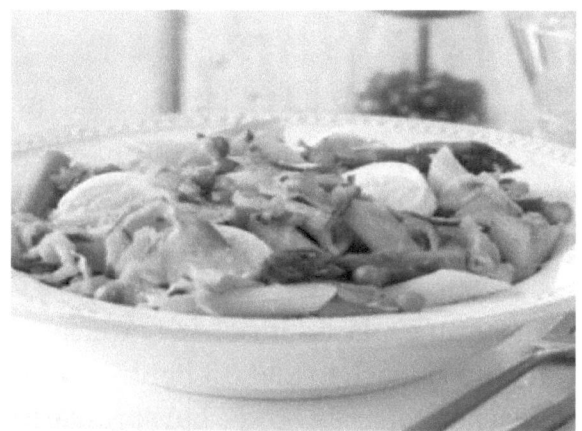

This pasta meal is really healthy with vegetable and chicken. Addition of egg on the top of pasta will increase their taste and flavor.

Serves: 4
Preparation Time: 35 minutes

Ingredients

- 500 ml chicken stock
- 250 g rice (long grain)
- 300 g turkey (cooked and diced)
- 250 g baby spinach
- 2 shredded carrot
- 1 teaspoon sesame oil (toasted)
- 1 teaspoon sesame seed (toasted)
- 2 tablespoons vegetable oil
- 4 eggs

- 2 tablespoons chili sauce

Method

1. Take a large pan and pour chicken stock in it. Let this stock boil and add the chicken and pasta into it. Let it boil again and cook for almost 12 to 15 minutes. Put rice and turkey in a bowl and keep it aside.

2. In the meantime, place spinach in one colander and pour hot water on spinach to make it lightly wilt. Keep carrots and spinach in separate bowls, but sprinkle sesame seeds and oil on both bowls.

3. Cover your cooked rice and keep them aside. Take a cooking pan and heat some vegetable oil on high heat. Fry eggs to make them crispy and roughly round.

4. Take serving bowls and spoon rice into bowls. Arrange carrots and spinach on the top. Top each bowl with chilli sauce and fried eggs. Serve hot!

18. Mexican Huevos Rancheros

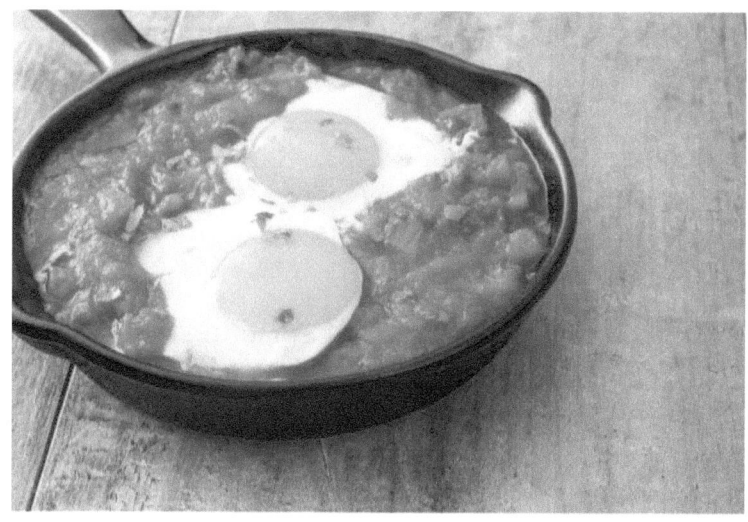

Fun Fact: Huevos Rancheros means Ranch Eggs

Prep Time: 20 mins.
Serves: 4

Ingredients

- 8 pastured eggs
- 1 medium onion
- 2 large tomatoes, chopped
- 3 Anaheim Chilies
- ½ tsp cumin
- ½ tsp chili powder
- 1 tsp adobo sauce
- 2 tsp sea salt
- Ghee

- Extra Virgin Olive Oil

Method

1. Heat 2 tablespoons ghee in large frying pan. Add onion, sauté until translucent. Add chilies, sauté for a minute. Add tomatoes, cumin, adobo, chili and sea salt. Cover and simmer on low for 15 mins.

2. In a frying pan set over medium heat, add two tablespoons of ghee. Drop each egg individually into the pan and fry until egg yolks are set as you like. Plate sauce, top with fried eggs and serve.

19. Menemen aka Istanbul's Breakfast

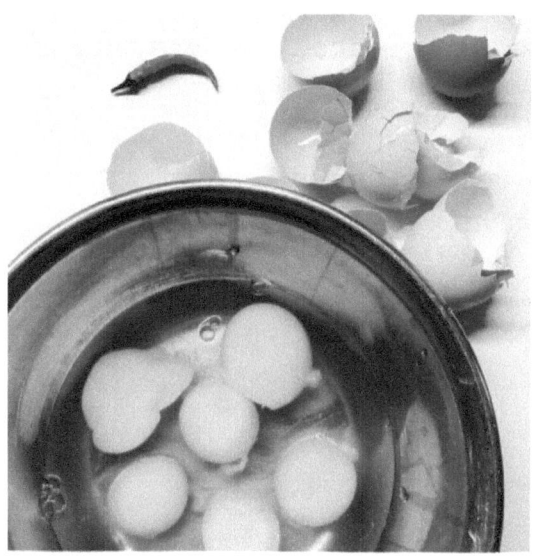

Prep Time: 15 mins.
Serves: 4

Ingredients

- 8 pastured eggs
- 4 large tomatoes, finely-diced
- 1 green bell pepper, finely-diced
- ¾ tsp sea salt
- ½ tsp oregano
- ½ tsp red pepper flakes
- Extra virgin olive oil
- 2 medium cucumbers, sliced

Method

1. Pour 2 tablespoons of olive oil in a frying pan, add salt, oregano, pepper flakes and bell pepper, and cook for a minute. Add tomatoes, cook for 5 minutes on low.

2. Whisk pastured eggs in bowl, pour over tomatoes and gently mix. Cook for two minutes and serve with tomato and cucumber.

20. Tuscany Pastured Eggs

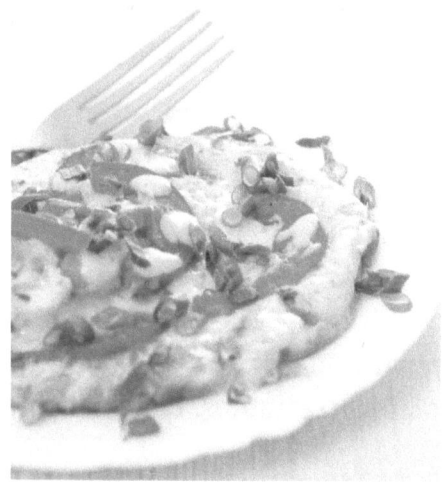

Serves: 4
Prep Time: 10 mins.

Ingredients

- 6 pastured eggs
- 6 cups of wild mushrooms
- 2 green bell peppers, seeded, julienned
- 1 large tomato, finely-chopped
- 2 green onions, finely-chopped
- ½ cup black olives, pitted
- 1/2 cup roasted red peppers
- ½ cup almonds, crushed
- ½ tsp sea salt
- ½ tsp black pepper
- Extra virgin olive oil

Method

1. Whisk pastured eggs with salt and black pepper, set aside. Pour 3 tablespoons of olive oil in a medium pot.

2. Add onions and sauté for a minute or until translucent. Add olives and red peppers and almonds, sauté for two minutes.

3. Top with pastured eggs, cover with your big tomato, green peppers and drizzle with olive oil. Turn to low and cover, cook for 10 minutes. Plate and enjoy hot.

21. Chinese Egg Drop Soup

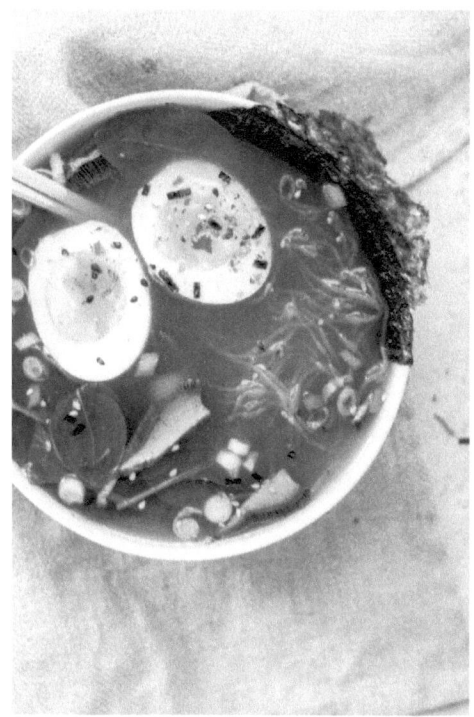

Prep Time: 10 mins.
Serves: 4

Ingredients

- 6 cups low-sodium chicken broth
- 4 pastured eggs
- 2 scallions, finely-chopped
- Sea Salt
- Black pepper

Method

1. Whisk your eggs in a bowl. Place chicken broth and scallions in a pot on medium heat and bring to a simmer.

2. Using a fork, drop swirls of whisked eggs into broth so you get ribbons.

3. Once you've added all the eggs, remove from heat and serve immediately. Add salt and pepper to your taste.

22. Avocado Egg Salad

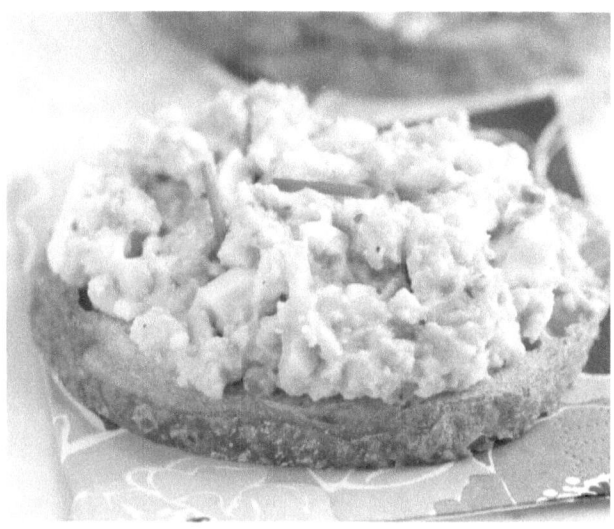

This egg salad that is made without mayo and has avocado in it instead.

Serving size: 2
Overall time: 30m

Ingredients

- Hard boiled eggs (4, chopped)
- Avocado (1/2, peeled and diced)
- Readymade mustard (2 tablespoons)
- Celery (2 stalks, finely chopped)
- Salt (1 teaspoon)
- Black pepper (1 teaspoon)
- Garlic powder (1 teaspoon)

Method

1. Place all ingredients in a large bowl and mix until thoroughly combined. Serve and enjoy.

23. Hummus Egg Salad

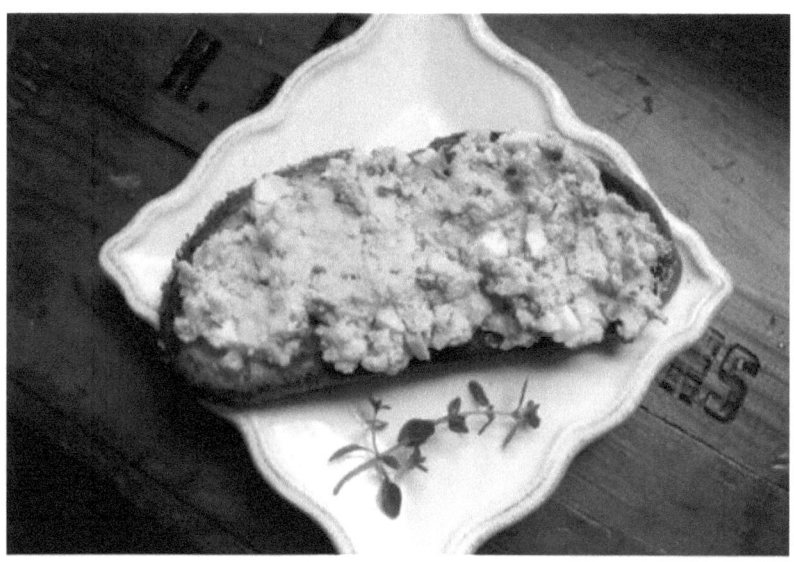

This egg salad is made with hummus, so it does not have any mayo or any dressing.

Serving size: 1
Overall time: 2h10m

Ingredients

- Hard boiled eggs (3, chopped)
- Hummus (3 tablespoons)
- Celery seed (1 pinch)
- Hot pepper sauce (1 dash, optional)
- Salt and black pepper (to taste)

Method

1. Place all ingredients in a large bowl and mix until completely combined.

2. Chill for 2 hours or more in a refrigerator. Serve and enjoy.

24. Pork Egg Salad

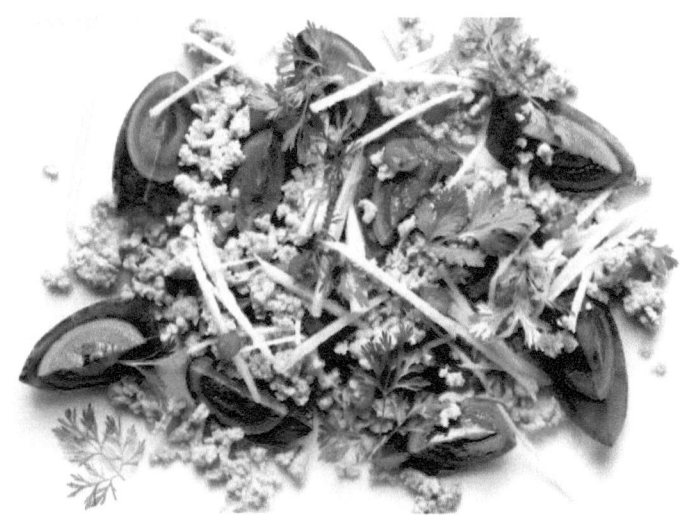

If you love ground pork, then you will love this egg salad recipe.

Serving size: 2
Overall time: 45m

Ingredients

- Hard boiled eggs (4, chopped)
- Ground pork (1/3 pound, cooked)
- Fresh ginger (1 peeled knob, julienned)
- Fish sauce (3 tablespoons)
- Lime juice (5 tablespoons)
- Sugar (1/2 teaspoon)
- Cilantro leaves (a few)

Method

1. Place all ingredients in a large bowl and mix until completely combined. Serve and enjoy.

25. Beef Egg Salad

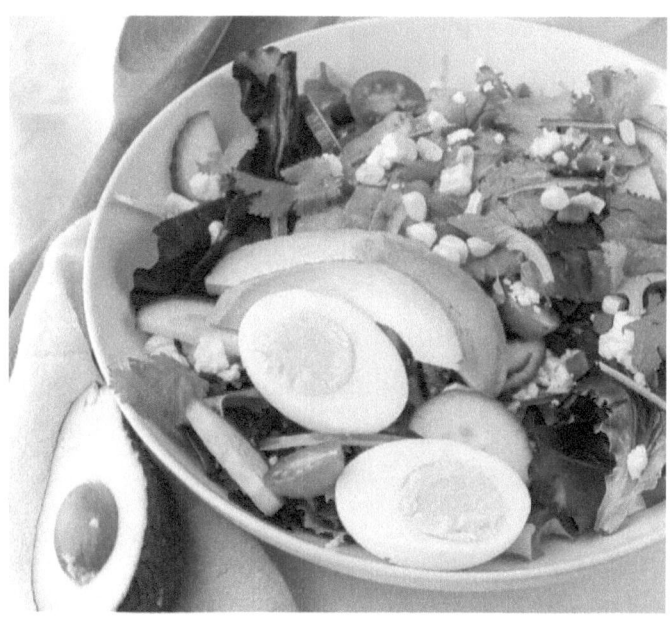

For all those beef lovers, you can try this combination of beef with egg salad.

Serving size: 4
Overall time: 45m

Ingredients

- Hard boiled eggs (4, chopped)
- Skirt steak (3/4 pound, cooked)
- Romaine lettuce (1 head, separated leaves)
- Radicchio (1 head, separated leaves)
- Tomatoes (1 pound, cut into wedges)
- Red onion (1 small, thinly sliced)

- Extra- virgin olive oil (3 tablespoons)
- Sherry or red wine vinegar (2 tablespoons)
- Salt and black pepper (to taste)

Method

1. Season the steak with black pepper and salt. Then cook to medium rare. Once done, let it rest for 5 minutes and cut against the grain.

2. Divide the lettuce, radicchio, tomatoes, steak, onion, and the eggs into four plates. Whisk the vinegar and the olive oil into a bowl.

3. Pour the dressing on each plate of salad. Serve and enjoy.

Final Words

I would like to thank you for downloading my book and I hope I have been able to help you and educate you about something new.

If you have enjoyed this book and would like to share your positive thoughts, could you please take 30 seconds of your time to go back and give me a review on my Amazon book page!

I greatly appreciate seeing these reviews because it helps me share my hard work!

Again, thank you and I wish you all the best with your cooking journey!

Disclaimer

This book and related site provides recipe and food advice in an informative and educational manner only, with information that is general in nature and that is not specific to you, the reader. The contents of this book and related site are intended to assist you and other readers in your personal efforts. Consult your physician or nutritionist regarding the applicability of any information provided in our information to you.

Nothing in this book should be construed as personal advice or diagnosis, and must not be used in this manner. The information provided about conditions is general in nature. This information does not cover all possible uses, actions, precautions, side-effects, or interactions of medicines, or medical procedures. The information in this site should not be considered as complete and does not cover all diseases, ailments, physical conditions, or their treatment.

No Warranties: The authors and publishers don't guarantee or warrant the quality, accuracy, completeness, timeliness, appropriateness or suitability of the information in this book, or of any product or services referenced by this site.

The information in this site is provided on an "as is" basis and the authors and publishers make no representations or warranties of any kind with respect to this information. This site may contain inaccuracies, typographical errors, or other errors.

Liability Disclaimer: The publishers, authors, and other parties involved in the creation, production, provision of information, or delivery of this site specifically disclaim any responsibility, and shall not be held liable for any damages, claims, injuries, losses, liabilities, costs, or obligations including any direct, indirect, special, incidental, or consequences damages (collectively known as "Damages") whatsoever and howsoever caused, arising out of, or in connection with the use or misuse of the site and the information contained within it, whether such Damages arise in contract, tort, negligence, equity, statute law, or by way of other legal theory.

www.ingramcontent.com/pod-product-compliance
Lightning Source LLC
Chambersburg PA
CBHW021132080526
44587CB00012B/1256